The Tibetan Book of the Dead for Beginners

Guidance & Preparation for Dying
By Lama Lhanang Rinpoche & Mordy Levine

"The past is history. The future is mystery.
The present moment is a gift."
—Lama Lhanang Rinpoche

The Tibetan Book of the Dead for Beginners

Published through -
Jigme Lingpa Center San Diego
PO Box 33231
San Diego, CA 92103
www.buddhistsandiego.com

All artwork created by Lama Lhanang

ISBN: 978-0-578-30911-8

May it be of benefit.

Dedication

May all beings have happiness and the causes of happiness.
May all beings be free from suffering and the causes of suffering.
May all beings rejoice in the wellbeing of others.
May all beings live in peace, free from greed and hatred.
                                        —The Four Immeasurables

We wish to express our great appreciation to those who helped this book come to fruition—Khandro Tsering Choeden, Maricruz Gomez, Alberto Garcia, Cynthia Orozco, Tom Seidman, Elizabeth Levine, Richard Harmon, Sondra Harmon, Catherine Stewart.

TABLE OF CONTENTS

Why this book?

In this day and age many people die suddenly, alone and with great emotional suffering for themselves and their family. As this book is being written, the Coronavirus pandemic rages in the years 2020 and 2021. Many people are dying in hospitals, alone, without the comfort of family, friends and loved ones by our side. Many appear to be ill prepared for the time of death.

The pandemic is also teaching us that it doesn't matter what our religion is, or our economic status or our viewpoints on any matter. In the end, we are all the same. No one wants suffering. We are all born. We will all die.

In most Western cultures, the topic of death comes in hushed voices. We shield our selves and our children from any meaningful discussion of death. Death is feared, and speaking of it creates discomfort. It is rarely discussed openly.

Western medicine and technology improve our health and can be lifesavers during critical times. Unfortunately, they are sometimes used to push death away, at the cost of unnecessary emotional suffering by the patient and family.

In Eastern cultures, senior citizens live within the community, and within the home of their family. As they age they are respected, supported and still a part of the community and family fabric. They live at home and die at home, in the bosom of their family and community.

Western culture tends to hide our seniors away in nursing homes or senior living centers—where we can visit them periodically. They are left to navigate the end of their lives with caretakers who fill in for family. Families rush in for the final lap. This is usually accompanied with fear, stress, great emotion and little sense of how to accommodate or support our loved one.

We are very fortunate that with the expansion of hospice care, our loved ones are dying with love and compassion. We can learn so much from the hospice care angels who care for our loved ones at the end of life.

Is it possible that death can be a celebratory empowering event? Is it possible to enjoy our lives and, as a result, be better prepared for death as it approaches? *What if death can truly become part of the cycle of life?*

Wouldn't it be best to understand what is going on as we, and our loved ones, age and die?

Buddhism, as practiced by Buddhists from the lineages of Tibetan Buddhism, is well equipped to prepare us for death. Buddhists know that how we live is how we will die. In Buddhism, daily practices, prayers, teachings and the prospect of death is used to motivate us to live an ethical and happy life. And living with joy and kindness, allows us to approach death with confidence and ease.

Death for Buddhists can be a smooth, natural and peaceful process, as we transition into our next post-life experience. To achieve this takes practice while we are alive, practice in the form of meditation, contemplation and skillful action while in this life, under the guidance of a qualified Buddhist Master.

If you study death, it can be a transforming, liberating event. If you don't, it can be very difficult emotionally.

The *Tibetan Book of the Dead*, as stated by scholars, was to have been composed in the 8th century by the great Buddhist Master Padmasambhava and then discovered in central Tibet in the 14th century. The text describes practices that prepare the advanced Buddhist practitioner for the experience that awaits us from the time we start to die until we are reborn. As one becomes more accomplished in this preparation, our level of confidence while alive and as we prepare for death increases. Through these practices, we also experience a sense of calm, compassion and wisdom.

When we are able to include the practices described by this great master in our daily lives, the prospect of death can be viewed as an empowering opportunity. A brief summary of the *Tibetan Book of the Dead* can be found in the Appendix.

Here are the The Dalai Lama's thoughts on death:

"As a Buddhist, I view death as a normal process, a reality that I accept will occur as long as I remain in this earthly existence. Knowing that I cannot escape it, I see no point in worrying about it. I tend to think of death as being like changing your clothes when they are old and worn out, rather than as some final end. Yet death is unpredictable: We do not know when or how it will take place. So it is only sensible to take certain precautions before it actually happens.

"Even if you are a great runner, you cannot run away from death. You cannot stop death with your wealth, through your magic performances or recitation of mantras or even medicines. Therefore, it is wise to prepare for your death.

"From a Buddhist point of view, the actual experience of death is very important. Although how or where we will be reborn is generally dependent on karmic forces, our state of mind at the time of death can influence the quality of our next rebirth. So at the moment of death, in spite of the great variety of karmas we have accumulated, if we make a special effort to generate a virtuous state of mind, we may strengthen and activate a virtuous karma, and so bring about a happy rebirth."
—His Holiness the Dalai Lama in the Foreword to
The Tibetan Book of Living and Dying by Sogyal Rinpoche

We offer this beginner's book on Buddhist practices and teachings on life and death, based on the *Tibetan Book of the Dead*, so that anyone who is interested can achieve calmness and confidence as death approaches them or a loved one.

And, as importantly, anyone can utilize these teachings to be happier while we are alive. This book is written to guide us to live our lives joyfully. The natural result will then be for us to die peacefully.

It is also our wish that this book will provide access to these precious teachings and practices to people of all religions. After all, in the events of life and death, we are all the same.

As the Dalai Lama says—

"When I see people with smiles, I feel these are all my brothers, sisters; seven billion human beings, actually, our brothers and sisters."

We hope this book is of great benefit to you and your loved ones.

How We Die

Case 1

Mom came to the intensive care unit 3 weeks ago in the middle of the night. Who could have predicted or prepared for this? Small and weak she is aware of her surroundings but unable to speak. She becomes weaker each day. From our conversations with her over the years we know her desire was to spend her last days at home. Now Mom is surrounded with beeping machines, tubes and medical personnel. She is hooked up to machines, without which she would certainly not live. We all know her days are numbered. We want to make sure that she dies peacefully without any physical or emotional pain. How can we do that now?

Case 2

My husband had been keeping himself alive for years despite his prognosis—with medication, meditation and gentle exercise. Death, once years away, had crept on us and became only weeks away. We slowed down our daily routines, and switched gears to make sure my husband would pass away in peace and quiet, surrounded by loved ones, and the music and art he loved so much. One day, after we had finished a recitation of his favorite poetry, his eyes closed. We knew that wherever his spirit or consciousness went he was happy, content and with no regrets.

Case 3

Our sister always ran around at warp speed in everything she did. From a toddler until her 32nd birthday, she was determined to achieve and do everything she possibly could at breakneck speed—regardless of what was in front of her or was left in her wake. Her car accident was just an extension of how she led her life. One instant she was our sister, the live wire—and then she wasn't. We learned from the police report that she was conscious for a few hours before eventually dying from a severe concussion. We never had a chance to say goodbye, or tell her how much we loved her.

These cases are sobering. And if you haven't been with someone who is dying, we can assure you that living through these experiences is more intense and prolonged then you could ever imagine. This is reality.

CHAPTER 1

Karma—How we live is how we die

"If a man or woman speaks or acts with a pure thought, happiness follows, like a shadow that never leaves."

—*Buddha (Dammapadha)*

You don't need to be a Buddhist to believe in karma, also known as the Law of Cause & Effect.

How we speak or act at this moment determines our experience in the next moment. How we live today impacts how we live tomorrow, the next day, the next week, month, year—when you believe in rebirth, in our future lives.

If we love unconditionally, love will come to us. When the flower grows, the bees and butterflies all come and enjoy it. When we open our heart everyone wants to be near. When we close our heart, no one wants to be around us.

Karma does not lie and we can't run away from it. If we really want to know our karma, look at yourself in the mirror. How we are now results from what we have done in our life until now. Our karma in the future is determined by what we are thinking, talking and saying now.

How does the law of karma work?

Here are a few examples:

If we are generous with someone then three consequences may follow:

1. we will be generous again in the future (habitual consequence)
2. we will find ourselves in an environment where people are generous (environmental consequence)
3. we will be the recipient of someone else's generosity in the future (personal consequence)

If right now our colleague or loved one speaks to us in a way that triggers our anger, then these three consequences may follow:

1. we will be angry in a similar situation in the future
2. we will find our self in an environment where those around us are angry
3. we will find our self in a situation where others are angry with us

Every thought, speech or action that we take as a reaction to what happens to us or around us, creates karma, a consequence.

Our intention precedes or triggers our thoughts, speech or actions. Intention is the basis of karma. Good intention yields good karma, and vice versa.

As we change our inner world—through thought, speech and action—the external world around us reflects those changes.

When does one experience the results of one's action? When does karma come to fruition?

From here on when we speak of *action* we refer to speech, physical action or thought.

We experience the 'fruits' of our actions anytime from the very next moment to years or lifetimes later.

Let's use the analogy of planting a vegetable seed in a field. When does it ripen? And how good will it taste?

Well, that depends on many variables. Here are just a few—sun, earth, fertilizer, water, how much sun, how much water, when was it watered, is it a big seed, is it a small seed, how many seeds, what was the ground like, what season was it planted, etc.

These are but a few of the variables that determine the result of the seed being planted.

Karma *seeds* that are in your mind, likewise, sometimes ripen immediately and sometimes in the future. The future for most Buddhists includes this lifetime, as well as future lifetimes.

From a Tibetan Buddhist lineage perspective, we also have the ability to purify our negative karma. Purification practices are an important focus of chanting and prayers in Tibetan schools of Buddhism. They include meditation, an admission or confession of the actions that created the negative karma, remorse and intention not to commit the actions that caused the negative karma again in the future.

And we can dilute our negative karma—just by doing more positive actions, and fewer actions that create negative karma.

As mentioned earlier, what we experience now in life is a result of all of our actions until this moment.

And likewise, how we deal with circumstances around us now determines our future. So, in a sense, from this moment on, we all create our own karma!

Our future is not predetermined. We determine it.

To quote the Buddha from the Dhammapada verse (276): "You yourselves must strive; the Buddhas only point the way."

We are planting karma *seeds* in our field of consciousness with every action we take, and those seeds mature at different rates, with different strengths and in different ways. Our intention, and the strength of it, is the basis of karma.

Also, we don't have a single independent karma account, like a bank account with a running balance.

We've got lots of karma accounts at different stages of development. All we can see at any one moment are the seeds that are currently sprouting. As for the other seeds that haven't yet sprouted, good—or bad—we can't see those at all. They sprout at different rates and times, and interact with each other, as well.

Once again, it is not just physical actions that create karma. Actions include those of the body, speech and thoughts.

If our intentions are full of friendliness, that will generate good karma. If our mind's intentions are selfish and full of pride, then that will generate negative karma.

We develop habits of body, speech and mind that we continue to reinforce—until we break the habit.

Each day we continue with our habits, reinforces the habit the next day. If we are a generous kind person today—and create a habit of these actions, those habits are stay with us tomorrow and the next day. That chain reaction continues until the moment we die—and, as we shall see, after death as well.

The key to transforming our life is what we do in this moment—now.

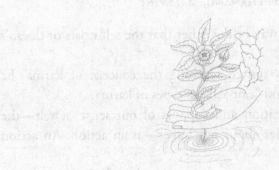

CHAPTER 2

What dies and what gets reborn?

Does our body die? Clearly.

What about our brain? That clearly dies too.

What about our personality, our soul, our spirit, our identity, our sense of self?

Before we talk about death and rebirth, we need to know what is dying. And for those who believe in rebirth, what is getting reborn.

Lets start by examining this thing that we call the "self"?

Here is a working definition of the self.

The self is who we think we are, based on the stories we tell our selves. We develop, nurture, protect and prop up our identity with stories about our selves and the world around us.

A common question in Buddhism, and many religions and philosophies, is 'does the self exist'?

And the Buddhist answer is 'Yes it does, but not in the way we think or act'.

The self is not a permanent solid "I" or "me". It is a constantly changing sense of who we think we are—from moment to moment and from day to day. It is not a fixed concrete entity.

Many religions believe in a soul—a permanent, eternal, unchanging, underlying essence. Buddhism does not. In fact, the Buddha himself never said one way or the other that the self exists or doesn't exist.

When the Buddha started teaching the concept of karma, he viewed ideas of "self" and "not-self" as types of karma.

He defined the creation and support of our sense of self—the habitual telling of stories about our selves—as an action. An action creates karma.

Being generous is an action that creates karma. Being mean or cruel creates karma. Likewise, how we develop our identity or sense of self—is karma that we create as well.

The question becomes, under what circumstances does the action of developing your "self" create positive or negative karma.

Here are 3 examples:

Example 1

John views himself as a good father and a good husband. He is convinced that he is and takes great pride in himself. The stories that he tells himself about being a good father or husband support that aspect of his self-identity.

But his wife and son do not see him as a good father or a good husband after he yells at them. This creates an ongoing conflict in the family, with all family members holding onto their views strongly.

The more John grasps and holds onto the concept that he is a good father or husband, the more negative karma he creates. If John is open-minded about who he thinks he is, and is able to consider other perspectives in this regard, creates positive karma.

The degree of grasping and attachment of John's 'self' determines whether he creates positive or negative karma. The judging and grasping of his self, and stories he tells himself, creates negative karma.

Example 2

Susan has her dream job as a surgeon in a hospital, where she has worked for 10 years. She loves it. It is part of her being. The strong view of her self is intertwined with her career as a surgeon. In the medical field, many doctors or nurses see their occupation as a "calling".

One day, Susan visited a patient after surgery and was very abrupt in her manner. Her patient was very upset and told others that Susan was a horrible physician. Susan was extremely upset and angry. Her patient's view was in direct conflict with the strong beliefs Susan had of herself and identity.

If Susan was open to the possibility that she was not the best physician she could have been at that moment, she is creating positive karma. If Susan is absolutely 100% sure that everything she did was perfect and leaves no room for improvement, that would create negative karma.

The grasping to support a strong sense of self-identity creates negative karma. Considering alternative views of the self loosens that grasping of self-identity, and creates positive karma.

Example 3

Joe is nervous in social environments, and it causes him anxiety. Joe tells himself stories (true or false) over and over again about how he thinks he is (or should be) in social environments. The action of creating these stories support his view of himself.

The more Joe believes the self-dialogue of "I am a shy, private person that doesn't do well around people", the more he is grasping to his sense of self.

The more Joe grasps, the more resistance arises when it is time to go to, or avoid, social engagements. This is an example of negative karma being created.

The degree of conflict Joe feels, or the stronger his reaction is to what happens around him—is a reflection of how strong his sense of self is.

Example 4

Mary is afraid of heights but continues to work on reducing that fear. By doing so, Mary weakens her sense of self, and moves away from identifying herself as someone who is afraid. This is an example of creating positive karma.

If Mary didn't work on that fear, or let it continue or worsen, that strengthens her identity, in this regard. This is an example of creating negative karma.

And of course, this aspect of Mary's self-identity is formed and strengthened by the myriad of stories that she tells herself about this fear.

Summary

How we view and strengthen (or weaken) our sense of self—is a type of karma that is created.

We can measure the degree of grasping we have when we look at how strong our tendencies or habits are.

We can measure how strong these habits are by how much internal resistance we feel when something happens that doesn't fit our view of our self.

Look at how we react to what happens to us or around us. A strong reaction to support our sense of self creates negative karma.

Look at the triggers that create a negative state of mind. A strong reaction to those triggers is indicative of the increased attachment to our self-identity. The stronger we support our self-identity, the greater the negative karma.

The good news is, since we create our self and our habits, we can also control it.

What is the answer to the question—'what gets reborn'?

What is reborn is our consciousness that contains our karmic impressions, or our ingrained habits. The karmic seeds we create are like impressions in our consciousness, a type of memory.

Our consciousness contains our sense of self. It is a type of memory or impression that continues on after we die.

Here are some common situations when we grasp and tell ourselves stories to support our identity—which creates karma. How much we judge ourselves or hold onto our perspective, determines whether the karma we create is negative or positive.

- Fear of heights
- Attachment to money
- Grasping at fame
- Self-importance
- Aversion to social engagements
- Fear of failure
- Fear of intimacy

How we grasp (or not) in these situations create impressions that get strengthened (negative karma) or weakened (positive karma) in our consciousness.

The consciousness containing these impressions is what continues on after our body and brain dies—and eventually is reborn in a new body.

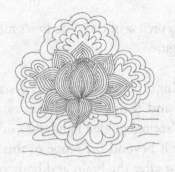

CHAPTER 3

Where does our consciousness go after death?

When we die our physical body returns to nature. Death is a natural part of the cycle of life. We are born, so we must die.

Like a flower that grows into beauty; after it dies, its seeds grow continuing the flower's lifecycle. Similarly, after we die our consciousness continues onto its next phase.

As mentioned earlier, our habits (karma) are embedded in our consciousness and continue on.

Let's start with the immediate moments after death—defined medically as when the heart stops beating, which results in immediate cessation of brain activity.

There are numerous documented stories of people who have experienced death and come back to life within minutes. These are termed 'near death experiences' ("NDEs"). These people have shared their stories and experiences with the general public, and with scientists who have tested the veracity of their experience.

Common NDE experiences include:

- when the dead person hears and sees people as their consciousness floats above their body,
- sees light at the end of a tunnel,

- experiences a review of their lifetime's memories, or
- sees a god figure.

Many people who experience an NDE describe feeling a certain relief after they die and their consciousness exits their body. Many experiences include 'seeing' golden light and / or luminous beings.

And although it is beyond the scope of this book to detail these NDEs, we know that after the brain and body cease to work, awareness continues, as documented in thousands of these cases.

In addition to these profound experiences, great saints and meditation masters of many faiths tell of their consciousness maintaining awareness after their body has been dead for days, and in some cases weeks.

What about the vast majority of those who die and do not return to their body, those who remain dead? From a Buddhist perspective, the consciousness experiences an intermediate, transition-like state until it is reborn in a new body.

The experiences in this state, or period of time until rebirth, are known as the Intermediate State, or the *bardo*. The English translation for the bardo appropriately enough is 'gap'.

The Tibetan Book of the Dead, which has inspired this book, describes what happens to us when we die. It also details what we can do to improve our experience in the bardo, and prepare us for a good rebirth.

Bardo can also refer to any gap in one's life. For example, the term bardo can be used to refer to a pause in between breaths, a vacation, a pandemic year, a time of change or transition.

Tibetan Buddhist lineages map our lifecycle in terms of 6 bardos (time periods), as follows:

1. The time period of our lives as we are experiencing it now.

2. The time period when we are asleep and dreaming.

3. The time period when we are meditating.

The last 3 bardos refer to the time periods between death and rebirth. The English translation of the Tibetan names are used here:

4. *Bardo of Dying*—This refers to the time period when our body is in the process of dying. All the elements of our body dissolve, and only pure awareness remains. During this period our mind can become very clear, and can recall all of our past positive and negative actions that we have done. We feel at peace as we remember the positive actions, and fearful, as we recall the negative actions.

5 *Bardo of Luminosity*—We experience visionary and auditory experiences—not unlike the dream state while sleeping when we are alive. This can include the appearance of ghosts, demons, gods, as well as a judge of our karmic account—all created by our state of mind.

6. *Bardo of Becoming*—The time between from when our consciousness (karma) enters the mother's womb until the time we are reborn. Entry into the mother's womb results from the consciousness' habit of grasping for a physical body for its identity, or a sense of self.

Specifically for this book, the use of the word bardo will refer to the 4th, 5th and 6th bardos described above. Tibetan Buddhist lineages teach that our consciousness can be in the 5th bardo for up to 49 days.

While in the 5th bardo, we experience a variety of phenomena. Some of our experiences are very similar to the dream state we experience while asleep during this lifetime. During the dream state, we can experience happy dreams, nightmares and every kind of experience imaginable in between.

Buddhists teach that while we are asleep our dreams are a reflection of our state of mind. For example, if prior to going to sleep we watch a happy uplifting movie, we are more likely to have happy dreams. If prior to sleep we have a very difficult or stressful day at work, or an argument with a loved one, we are more likely to have a negative dream experience.

When we discussed karma, we saw that each moment impacts the next moment in our lives. Just as our moments prior to sleeping impact our dream state, our moments prior to death also impact our experience in the bardo.

Our dreams are also impacted by how we live our life as well. Our karmic tendencies impact our dreams as well. If we are angry, that will be reflected in our dreams, and vice versa. If we are constantly grasping for financial gain, power, sex or love, that tendency influences our experience in dreaming.

More specifically, dream yoga practitioners are individuals who practice awareness while dreaming, and are able to control their dream experience. The training for this skill includes meditation practices that enable us to control our states of mind when awake, as well as when asleep.

The skills practiced in dream yoga help the practitioner navigate and influence the experience in the 5th bardo, the *Bardo of Luminosity*. We will discuss some of these meditation practices in the next chapters.

How we live our life—the karma we create—determines our state of mind prior to death, our experience in the bardo, and our rebirth.

When we die, as mentioned earlier, our karmic habits, embedded in our consciousness, continue into the bardo. The degree of grasping and attachment, to maintain our self-importance, plays center stage for our consciousness in the bardo.

If we live our lives with the aim to reduce our grasping and our fears, being kind to others, understanding that life is impermanent; then those efforts will be reflected positively in our consciousness as we enter the bardo. Our experiences in the bardo will not be nightmarish.

Our state of mind in the bardo similarly impacts the kind of rebirth we will have. One moment impacts the next—regardless of where we are in our continuum of the birth-life-death-rebirth cycle.

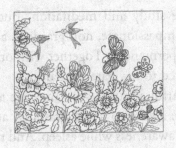

CHAPTER 4

How can we influence our next rebirth?

Will we be reborn in a 'good' family? Will we be reborn in a well to do city, or a poor desolate neighborhood or country? Will we be reborn as a human or an animal?

Great Buddhist masters who have trained over many years (or lifetimes) are able to choose their family and location of rebirth. In fact, before they die, many masters will go so far as to leave a letter and other information for their students as to where they will be reborn. This allows their students to find them after rebirth. The students search with the clues provided by their teacher. When they find a candidate who might be the rebirth of their teacher, they test a young child in a variety of ways, to be certain the child is their former teacher. The child can now 'continue' their Buddhist studies, and continue to work reduce suffering for all sentient beings.

An inspiring movie to watch this take place is Unmistaken Child. A Buddhist monk, Tenzin Zopa, is tasked with finding his teacher Geshe Lama Konchog, in his new incarnation.

The most well known example of this cycle is the life of His Holiness the Dalai Lama XIV. As a child, he was identified, tested and found to be the prior incarnation of His Holiness the Dalai Lama XIII.

Through intense study and meditation, Buddhist masters train their minds to be compassionate, non-grasping, and truly understand that the world is impermanent. Together with other advanced teachings, they are prepared to navigate the bardo.

They are not fearful about death. They are able to control their states of mind while awake to avoid grasping, attachment and fear. They maintain their awareness while asleep. And they are able to navigate the bardo with stability and awareness—the same way they lived their lives.

Great masters approach death the same way they live—with compassion for themselves and others. They have ceased, or reduced, their grasping of their "self".

Likewise for us, how we live is how we will die. How we die is how we will experience the bardo. How we experience the bardo will be one of the ingredients that determine how and where we are reborn.

For most of us, we are not able to control our states of mind while awake or asleep. We grasp at the people, events and things that are around us, and become attached to our desire or aversion to them. When our situation changes in a way we don't like, we experience stress, anger, annoyance or irritation.

When we have good experiences, bad experiences or nightmares, it seems like these things just happen to us. And we react based on our prior habitual reactions. We don't have the ability to control our reactive state of mind.

And if we are not able to control our minds during our waking hours, we will certainly not be able to be aware of, or control, our minds when we sleep, or are in the bardo.

The way we live our life—which includes our level of awareness, degree of grasping, and other tendencies—is how we will experience the bardo. It is very important to be able to 'let go' of our reactive grasping tendencies when in the bardo.

In addition, the bardo experience is more difficult to navigate than the normal dream state we experience while alive.

For most of us, death can be a big shock to our consciousness, especially when it is sudden.

After death many beings enter the bardo in a state of shock and resist the fact that they are dead. Good examples of this are the movies Sixth Sense (starring Bruce Willis), or the movie Ghost (with Patrick Swayze, Demi Moore, and Whoopi Goldberg).

Some recently deceased cling to their former lives. Even while dead, they are aware of their family and friends who are still living and going about their lives. If family and friends are agitated or arguing during or after the death event, that will impact consciousness of our loved one in the bardo—and create agitation for the consciousness. If friends and family are able to maintain a sense of calm, peace and love, that will allow the deceased to be at peace while the deceased continues through the bardo.

Consciousness experiences the bardo without a physical body.

While alive, our physical body is very grounding for us.

When we get out of bed in the morning or when we exercise, our physical body grounds us and helps our state of mind stabilize. For example, if we are stressed, we can take a walk or exercise our physical body. This helps to clear the physical, emotional and psychological stress. Our mind–body connection is strong. What effects one impacts the other seamlessly.

When we meditate and observe our breath, we also connect our mind to our body.

While alive, our physical body in partnership with our mind interacts with the physical world around us, which is also grounding.

In the bardo we don't have our physical body to support us. We only have our consciousness—untethered from the body.

As mentioned earlier, in the bardo our consciousness includes our karma, the habits and tendencies that we have created, developed and maintained through our lifetime(s).

If we are not able to control our states of mind while we are alive in our body, imagine how difficult it is after we die—when the mind is untethered from our physical body.

As we can see, navigating the bardo without preparation can be difficult. Our state of mind in the bardo mirrors our state of mind in this lifetime; without a body and in many cases in shock.

If we spent our lives grasping at desire and aversion, then the grasping to avoid fear and seeking for pleasure and comfort will play out in our experience in the bardo.

As mentioned in the previous chapter, at the end of the *Bardo of Luminosity* the grasping momentum of the consciousness, usually within 49 days, seeks to be in a body again. It seeks a womb, a physical body. And based on its karma, consciousness finds and enters a womb.

Karma determines our place of birth, family, location of birth, etc. For most beings, at this time in the cycle of life-death-rebirth, there is very little choice as to our rebirth environment. It is determined by our karma.

Can we prepare for the bardo—now that we know how much is riding on it?

We would all prefer to have a pleasant experience as we experience dying. If we know the bardo experience is going to be unpleasant—or we are unprepared—we would be living our lives in fear, and die in fear.

Appropriate preparation allows us to mentally relax to some degree. When we know what to expect and prepare our minds, we will feel more confident and peaceful as we approach the bardo.

Finally, from a very practical perspective, how we live our lives, including how we experience the bardo, determines our rebirth. Will you be reborn in a peace-loving family or an uncaring family? Will you be reborn as an animal or a calm human? Let's prepare now while we can.

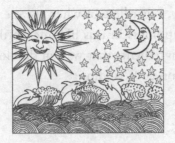

CHAPTER 5

Start where we are now

Buddhist practitioners study, contemplate and meditate to train their state of mind to be more compassionate (with our self and with others) and to see reality as it truly is, always changing.

Regardless of what transpires in life, we know that our state of mind is:

- the only thing we can control, and
- the key to leading a happy life free of suffering.

Buddhist practitioners train their mind to reduce fear and grasping (which creates good karma), and to develop compassion for others (which reduces our permanent sense of self).

Mind training, through meditation, study and prayer, reduces our suffering and improves our state of mind in this lifetime. At the same time, these activities help us prepare for the bardo experience when we die.

As we polish our mind to improve our experience in our current lifetime, our experience as we approach death, and in the bardo, will automatically improve.

25

More specifically, regardless of when we die, there are two critical ingredients to happiness in this lifetime, in the bardo and future lifetimes. The two ingredients that we can develop and realize in our minds are Compassion & Wisdom.

Compassion

From a Buddhist perspective, we do our best to develop compassion—actualized as the desire to reduce suffering for all beings. We learn to develop compassion for ourselves and for others—regardless of who they are and whether we like them or not. And yes, that includes people or sentient beings we don't like!

How does this help us? As we develop compassion for others, we reduce our grasping and support of our own ego. They are two sides of the same coin.

When our mind looks at our situations with a focus on how it impacts upon 'me' and 'I', we automatically view ourselves as separate from others. We note differences, and create judgments based on 'me' versus 'other'. This mindset increases the grasping and support of our self-identity. And we know, that as the grasping and support of our ego increases, we increase negative karma. More plainly, when our focus is primarily on ourselves, long term inner happiness will never be ours.

Developing compassion creates good karma, reduces our sense of separateness and in a direct sense we also feel better about ourselves. The impact of 'me' and 'I' thinking is weakened. In fact, our natural state of being contains a strong sense of compassion for others, as well as ourselves.

The Dalai Lama has spoken extensively about this topic:

"When we feel love and kindness toward others, it not only makes others feel loved and cared for, but it helps us also to develop inner happiness and peace."

"If you want others to be happy, practice compassion. If you want to be happy, practice compassion."

Developing a mind of compassion is a critical ingredient to our own happiness in this life. A mind of compassion is also a critical ingredient for when we experience the Bardo of Dying, Bardo of Luminosity and Bardo of Becoming.

To paraphrase one Lama—when you develop compassion in this lifetime, it is as if the universe rolls out the red carpet when you enter the bardo.

Practice Developing Compassion

There are many ways to develop Compassion. One simple way is to recite, meditate or contemplate a prayer called the *4 Immeasurables*.

The *4 Immeasurables* describes 4 attributes that we can develop for our self and others: loving-kindness, compassion, joy and equanimity.

The prayer can be repeated numerous times as we contemplate its meaning:

"May all beings have happiness and the causes of happiness.
May all beings be free from suffering and the causes of suffering.
May all beings rejoice in the wellbeing of others.
May all beings live in peace, free from greed and hatred."

Line by line, it can be interpreted as follows:

- Loving-kindness is the desire that all of us are friendly toward each other and wish them well.
- Compassion is the desire that all beings, including our selves, not suffer.
- Joy is being happy for others' happiness and success.
- Equanimity means not being strongly attached to things we like, or strongly averse to things we don't like. We develop equanimity when we reduce our aversions and desires and strive to keep an even emotional keel. After all, everything always changes, so why grasp at something so strongly that inevitably will change.

We can also reflect on the prayer's meaning and study it until over time, little by little, we can feel it in our minds and live it in our lives.

Initially, while we repeat this prayer, we can hold our self and loved ones in our mind.

Over time, while we recite the prayer, we might incorporate those who we feel neutral about in our minds.

And eventually, while we recite the prayer, we might consider bringing into our mind people who we may not like, or have not treated us well.

People err or make mistakes. We err and make mistakes. We certainly do not condone bad behavior. However, many people behave and act poorly as a result of an upbringing of abuse, or an environment which contributes to their behavior. We cannot pretend to know others' motivation when they cause harm or insult.

We do not condone their behavior, and we also do not wish suffering on them. By wishing harm on others—we harm ourselves and develop negative karma by doing so.

This shift in how we view others and ourselves moves us closer and closer to a life with reduced ego, less stress and greater happiness. Grudges are forgotten, self-talk about the past or future—what 'should have' or 'might have' been—fades. This leaves us with a life enjoying and experiencing the present moment, as is.

The past is history, the future is mystery and the present moment is a gift.

The development of compassion leads to a more peaceful death—a death with less worry, less stress, a better experience in the bardo, and eventually, a more auspicious rebirth.

Additional practices that can incorporate a mind of compassion into our daily lives are found in the Appendix.

Wisdom of Realizing Impermanence and Emptiness

Understanding wisdom is the second key ingredient to living a happy life. The development of this type of wisdom also ensures a better experience in the bardo and future lifetimes.

Wisdom, in this case, means seeing reality accurately—without illusions.

In this case, emptiness refers to our sense of self. We asked earlier does our self exist? Yes and no. It exists—but not in the way we think. It is constantly changing and evolving. It does not have any permanent existence. We therefore say that the 'self' is empty of inherent existence. This realization over time helps us reduce our grasping and support of a solid self-identity—which is synonymous with being—and feeling free and liberated.

Understanding impermanence is the realization that everything around us—people, things and situations—changes. Nothing is permanent. This understanding also helps us to reduce our grasping—after all there is nothing solid to grasp onto. Grasping at something that isn't there causes us suffering when reality splashes water in our face—and we find out we were chasing an illusion.

Impermanence also allows us to see how we are all interrelated. Change happens when something *causes* it to happen. Change does not happen *independently* of anything. The Law of Cause and Effect, karma, is another way of experiencing how we are all dependent and related to each other. All that happens to us is a result of something or someone.

Thich Nhat Hanh, the great Zen master, calls this phenomena "*interbeing*". As he so eloquently describes it:

"Emptiness does not mean nothingness. Saying that we are empty does not mean that we do not exist. No matter if something is full or empty, that thing clearly needs to be there in the first place. When we say a cup is empty, the cup must be there in order to be empty. When we say that we are empty, it means that we must be there in order to be empty of a permanent, separate self.

About thirty years ago, I was looking for an English word to describe our deep interconnection with everything else. I liked the word "togetherness," but I finally came up with the word "interbeing." The verb "to be" can be misleading, because we cannot be by ourselves, alone. "To be" is always to "inter-be." If we combine the prefix "inter" with the verb "to be," we have a new verb, "inter-be." To inter-be and the action of interbeing reflects reality more accurately. We inter-are with one another and with all life."

The realizations of emptiness and impermanence are critical ingredients to our own happiness in this life. A mind that understands emptiness and impermanence on a day-to-day basis is a critical ingredient for:

- the time period approaching our death (the bardo of this lifetime),
- as we die (the bardo of dying) and
- as we travel through the bardo of luminosity.

Practice Developing Wisdom

Contemplating the impermanent nature of our life, our body, our environment, friends, loved ones and our possessions helps to reduce our grasping nature. The more we are able to reduce our grasping to what is impermanent, the happier our life will be, and the easier our death will be.

Meditation on our breath can help our mind to absorb the impermanence of our world. We can observe our breath as it rises and falls, comes and goes and changes from one moment to another. A sitting meditation that observes our breath in this manner helps develop the realization of emptiness and impermanence.

Observing our breath, and all of its uniqueness and observing our thoughts passing through our minds helps us to see that everything is always changing. And that's reality, and that's ok.

With eyes closed, spine tall (lying down is ok if sitting is uncomfortable or painful) and relaxed body, we simply observe our natural breathing. As we inhale we observe the air coming into our body. We can observe the air coming into our nose, or the rise of our abdomen. We can observe the air exiting through our nose or the gentle collapse in our abdomen.

When thoughts come into our mind and interrupt our observation—and they will—simply go back to observing our breathing, without any judgment whatsoever.

30

We play this 'game' of observing our breath, being interrupted and distracted, and going back to observing our breath. We can start with 10 minutes a day, and gradually over weeks, increase to 15-20 minutes a day. Maybe even twice a day!

With study, contemplation and meditation, over time, our mind calms and begins to accept the reality of emptiness and impermanence. Change is not bad or good. It just is. It does not mean that everything falls apart for the worse. Inevitable change simply means that everything is possible. As we realize this more and more, we are not surprised by change, and may even enjoy it. Ignorance of this reality is not bliss—only suffering.

Additional practices that we can incorporate into our daily lives to develop our understanding of wisdom are found in the Appendix.

How are Wisdom and Compassion related?

The more compassionate we become, the more positive karma we accumulate. We are reducing our grasping to our egos.

When we recognize that we all want to be happy and suffer as little as possible, we realize we are all the 'same'. This mindset reduces the 'me' versus 'other' separateness mentality.

Understanding the interrelated nature of everything is another way of understanding that nothing is permanent. We are connected to each other and dependent upon each other.

People like Mother Theresa and Mahatma Gandhi had such great compassion for others that they were also able to understand and see the emptiness and impermanence of everything.

Everything changes, and that is ok. This is normal—just like the law of gravity.

Conversely, when we understand impermanence and that everything is interdependent, this naturally leads to compassion for everyone. We understand that we are all interconnected. No borders really exist between you and me. There is no dualism. There is no 'you' over there and 'me' over here, no tribalism. In essence, we would have more of a sense of oneness.

As the Dalai Lama says: 'we are all brothers and sisters'.

Compassion leads to wisdom, and wisdom leads to compassion. Development of these two key ingredients leads us to a happier life, a peaceful death and an auspicious rebirth.

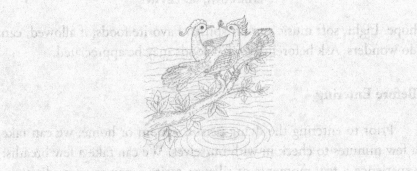

Chapter 6

How can we support our friends and loved ones as they approach death?

Our loved ones have lived their lives as best they can, and now their impending death awaits them. The past is gone, and can't be changed. And the final clock is ticking down. Maybe they believe in the bardo, maybe they don't. We can still help them die peacefully. These suggestions will help them transition without emotional suffering.

Prepare our State of Mind

Our loved one, and other visitors, may be in emotional and/or physical pain. We too may be in emotional pain as well. Sometimes that stress drives us to try and control what is going on around us. We think we know best. And we want to be of help. It is good to recognize that we are there to reduce suffering. We may not need to control anything. We can take the attitude of being of service to those who are suffering.

Plan ahead

Consider bringing a plant, flowers or pictures that might be enjoyed. Pictures made by children or grandchildren can bring joy and hope. Light, soft music can lift spirits. Favorite foods, if allowed, can do wonders. Ask beforehand what foods may be appreciated.

Before Entering

Prior to entering the dying person's room or home, we can take a few minutes to check in with ourselves. We can take a few breaths: experience a few moments of silence; recite a prayer or meditation. These will help us bring calm and love to our self and loved one.

Maintain a peaceful and quiet environment

As our loved ones are dying, they can be very sensitive, and their hearing can be quite good—regardless of their condition. Loud noises from another room, arguments and discussions about their condition, can all be understood and felt by them. Speaking quietly and calmly can allow them to feel at peace.

Limit or eliminate family tension

Any differences between family members should be placed on the backburner. Or better yet, now is a good time to mend any fences that may exist between family members or friends. Requesting, and giving forgiveness between people at this time, allows the dying person to let go when ready and be at peace.

Keep calm

The emotions you exhibit can be felt by those approaching death, and can impact their state of mind. If you are calm, they are more likely to be calm. If you are agitated or upset, it will be difficult for them to be calm. Remember, we want to afford them the opportunity to pass in a peaceful state of mind.

Be a good listener

Let's do our best to accommodate them. If they want to talk, then we can listen intently—without judgment. If they want quiet, we can offer peaceful silence. You can intuit what they might want—or just ask them. Even if they are not speaking, sitting in silence is a beautiful way to support and connect with another human being.

Offer specifics

You can ask them softly and gently if they want more water, ice chips, medication, food, or their favorite music. No need to bombard them with these questions. You can ask these questions a little at a time—gently and softly.

Do not push or pull

Be gentle. No need to pull or push them about any additional loose ends, tasks or things to think about. Now is not the time for decisions or weighty conversation.

Ensure they are physically comfortable.

Pillows, bed adjustments, bed direction, lights, sounds, or where you are sitting can all be sources of comfort or stress. Seek help if it is difficult to physically accommodate your friend or loved on. No rush. All may be done calmly and safely.

Music

Music can be helpful to calm the spirit. Offer to play their favorite music on a device, or directly from your voice to their ears. Sometimes the sound of the human voice in person can make a strong and supportive connection. Ask, or intuit what might make them feel comfortable.

Would they like any specific prayers recited or chanted

If possible, it's good to ask them in advance about this. But it is also ok to ask them what their preference is in that moment. Once again, their wishes are honored with respect. No judgment on anyone's part. Open mindedness and support are the watchwords of the time.

Surround them with a spiritual guide

Hang a picture of their favorite religious figure, saint or deity (e.g. Jesus, Moses, Buddha, Mary, etc.). If possible, it's good to ask in advance about this. But it is also ok to ask them what their preference is in that moment.

Be present

The best way to avoid feeling awkward, is just to be present. Observing and touching base with your natural breathing will help you stay present. A racing or agitated mind can settle through the observation of your natural breathing. Over-thinking about what you can, or should, do or say is not necessary. **Let it be.**

Regardless of their state of mind, we can be open and understanding. Most people are not prepared for dying. We can listen. Be present. Be calm.

Disagreements with family members or friends

Ask, or encourage the dying person to make up with anyone they may have had differences with. They can voice their sentiments or apologies to you, or do so silently. Their prayers will be heard. And of course, if requested, you will share their sentiments with the other party.

What may arise during the visit?

Your loved one can be experiencing fear, uncertainty, anger, guilt, regret, depression and a whole host of spiraling emotions.

If they want to hear your perspective, you can speak with a calm and reassuring tone and share:

- how they have done wonderful things in their life
- how their belief in God or other Higher Being will take care of them when they pass.
- that you will of course miss them. And you will remember all the wonderful memories you have; what you have learned, and what you will be able to pass onto others
- how their lives have impacted others for the better
- how much you or others have loved and cherished them
- how their presence in the world will live on through others, for generations to come.

Your loved one may appear not to be conscious of visitors or their surroundings.

Science has proven that people who are dying, or comatose, may in fact hear what is being said around them. With that in mind, we can still speak with them calmly, and express our love or respect or admiration for them.

How do you handle questions or concerns about God? Heaven and hell? An afterlife? The bardo?

In addition to the prior suggestions, you can assure your loved one that—

- God, or the Higher Presence that they believe in, is one of forgiveness and acceptance—and they can count on that.

37

- They can focus on their God, or a Higher Power that is always with them. That focus alone is enough to be welcomed into heaven, kingdom of God, the afterlife or bardo.
- Without any doubt their love, positive deeds and thoughts will do them well as they enter the next phase.

Repeating prayers or mantras, out loud or silently, will help them stay connected with God or that Higher Being. A mantra is a phrase or word whose sound and/or meaning resonate to help with concentration, or to clarify and purify our state of mind. Each faith has it's own phrases that can bring solace and comfort.

Christ, Mary, Buddha, the Prophet Mohammad and Moses are all representations and manifestations of love, compassion—a Higher Being. They can be relied on to hear anyone's call for help or compassion.

How can we recognize the signs of a natural death?

When we are attentive and our minds are clear, with some experience, we are able to see and feel the progression of the shutting down of the physical body.

By observing this progression we can know if death is near or still far off. Tibetan medicine has detailed the signs of the body's deterioration. They mirror closely to Western observations as well.

By studying what is going on in the body when it goes through the dying process, we will not be surprised as it happens. We can gain confidence or mental comfort as we follow this progression as it happens in others or ourselves. We can recite the appropriate prayers before death, and know when it is time to remove the body after death.

The following is a brief overview of the major signs that accompany the dying process:

Phase 1

The body feels weak, and feels like it is sinking into the earth. Eyes can't stay open, and the body's color is dull.

Phase 2

The body feels dry and one may feel very thirsty. The hearing sense is diminished.

Phase 3

Digestion is difficult. Memory fades. Inhalation is weak, while exhalation becomes relatively stronger. Smell is diminished or gone.

Phase 4

Awareness of what is going on is diminished. Taste is diminished or gone. Touch sense is diminished.

Phase 5

Gross consciousness ceases, subtle consciousness remains.

Phase 6—8

Wind energies gather at the heart chakra (center of the chest).

Depending upon one's preparation, the subtle mind may experience a state of clear light or the true nature of reality (for details, please see Appendix—Tibetan Book of the Dead—A Summary).

Consciousness leaves the body, which can be noted when the heart center is no longer warm. The body begins to smell as it decomposes. One has a subtle sense that the consciousness has left.

It is at this point, that traditional Buddhist Lamas recite prayers and have the body removed. In the absence of experienced Lamas, you may recite the prayers in next chapter.

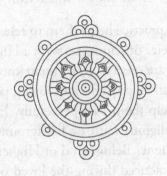

CHAPTER 7

What do Buddhist practitioners do as they are dying?

Buddhists from Tibetan lineages practice Phowa, a combination of visualization and mantra practice that transfers their consciousness, with all its karmic seeds, to a Higher Being, at the end of life.

Performing Phowa while dying reduces the burden of negative karma that the practitioner has accumulated through their lifetime(s).

When Phowa is performed with sincerity and surrender, the dying practitioner will have an auspicious rebirth in their next lifetime on earth. The dying practitioner who practices Phowa may have the option of attaining rebirth in a Pure Land. In that case, their consciousness would not be reborn in the world we currently live in.

A Pure Land is a land of beauty that exceeds all other worlds or realms that one can be reborn into. Being reborn into a Pure Land is equivalent to becoming enlightened.

Lamas from Tibetan Buddhist lineages may lead their dying students through the Phowa practice to help them attain an auspicious rebirth in the human realm, to reach the Pure Land, or to achieve enlightenment.

Dying Buddhist practitioners—as well as non-Buddhists—can practice a simplified, but effective, version of Phowa for themselves. And finally, you can lead your loved one through a version of Phowa practice, as well. The practice helps them to release grasping (negative karma), and unite their consciousness with a Higher Being.

If our loved ones are open to it, let them know you will lead them through a transformative, peaceful and loving practice, that will ease their suffering and help them pass peacefully. It can be practiced by anyone, from any religious faith or background. It will help them connect with their Higher Being, God or Higher Power.

Phowa may be practiced during the loved ones last living hours. We can guide them by reciting a short version of Phowa, provided below, with a soft, loving, and calm voice. Traditionally, it is recited with the guide sitting next to the loved one's head—not near their feet.

After we guide them several times, our loved one can practice this on their own as well.

In addition to Phowa, at the moment of death, we can also provide gentle encouragement to guide them on to the bardo, or world beyond. The encouragement will help them move forward, instead of clinging to their body or old life.

Here are examples of *Abbreviated Phowa Visualization* and *Encouragement* that we can recite to the dying person softly and slowly. If possible, sit physically close to them, and speak slowly and quietly into their ear.

Read the next section, filling in the Higher Presence or Supreme Being that they most relate to. This is best to do in advance. If you don't know, it is ok to ask them who that Higher Being might be: Jesus, Moses, Buddha, Mary, Mohammed, etc.

Abbreviated Phowa Visualization:
(Please feel free to modify as you see fit)

READ: Gently close your eyes and let's observe our breath for a few minutes.

Don't worry about any distracting thoughts or sounds that you may hear.

When you notice you are distracted, no problem. Just go back to observing your natural and unique breathing.

Observe the air coming in and out of your nostrils; or the rise and fall of your abdomen or chest. Just watch, and appreciate the breathing that has been your friend all of your life.

[Pause to allow them to observe their breath.]

READ: Imagine that your most precious God, Higher Presence or Golden Light is in the room.

It could be any Higher Being for whom you feel love or great respect, devotion or connection.

It does not matter whether or not you have had this connection during your lifetime. Now is all that matters.

We will be able to invoke their presence now.

[NAME OF HIGHER BEING->_____] has been with you all of your life, and now [circle one: he/she] is making [circle one: himself/herself] known to you.

Now is the time for you to imagine that [_____] is connected to your heart. [_____] has come to keep you company.

43

Imagine that [_____] is present in the form of a white light. That is all you need to feel now.

The warmth of the white light is around your head and flows from their into your heart. [_____]'s presence is calm and loving towards you.

You can feel [circle one: him/her]. And you can feel your sense of devotion to [him/her] coming from your heart.

[_____] is so happy to be with you and see you.

[_____] can feel your essence and you are very beautiful to [circle one: him/her].

[_____] is smiling at you and is so happy and appreciates you so much.

Take a few moments, or as long as you wish, so you can take in and feel their presence, and their white light.

It does not need to be any specific visualization; just a warm, loving sense of light.

[_____] has come to you to welcome you to your next phase.

Now, feel a similar light present in your heart center.

You too possess the same white light inside your heart center.

Take your time to appreciate, and welcome this moment and this feeling.

After you feel the same essence inside of you—feel a connection between your heart center and this beautiful Higher Being that is your guide, protector and loving presence.

Feel the connection. Now feel yourself and [_____] merge together into one essence.

You are coming home to be with them. They are so happy to be with you and welcome you.

Rest in that feeling for as long as you like.

Take your time. There is no rush. Repeat this whenever you would like.

Encouragement:

The following may be recited slowly and softly during the last moments of life. It is based on **Guru Padmasambhava's** teachings. Please feel free to modify as you see fit.

[Loved One's Name _____]

Do not be afraid. You are surrounded by love.

You have now arrived at the moment of death.

There is no turning back.

This is the natural state of the cycle of life for all living things.

Go forward to the [world beyond | the bardo].

Do not cling to the present life.

No need to grasp, or be attached to your previous life.

The body has expired.

It is time to move forward.

Take refuge in the presence of [NAME OF HIGHER BEING-> _____]

[Repeat the above several times and repeat the last line several times.]

CHAPTER 8

How can I help a dying loved one if I am not close by?

One can hold a loved one in mind—regardless of distance. It matters not where our friend, family member or loved one is. We can feel them. In our mind, we can see them. We can participate in any of these practices, prayers or visualizations—wherever we are and wherever they are.

We are all connected. We all affect each other—whether you feel it or not. When we look around and see all the numerous causes that create numerous consequences—we can't ignore that we are all connected.

The pandemic we are living in now is proof of that. We are no longer billions of individuals doing our own thing. We never were. We are not 195 countries existing independently in this world. The pandemic—as of this printing—has infected 213,000,000 people around the world. It went from one person to the next. Yes, we are all connected.

Suffering and love also traveled the distance. We can feel the suffering around the world. The images of suffering flashed around the world on TV, news or Internet is palpable.

We can feel the love for the families of those whose family members died and those who survived. We don't need to be in their living room to feel their pain or relief.

Many of us survived. Many of us helped others. Many countries supported individuals from countries on the other side of the world. There was a realization that we are all in this together.

As we pray, chant or visualize—do so as if our loved one is right next to you. They are. If you have any doubt, than 'try it on' and see what you feel. Practice the Phowa and the Encouragement provided above. Your loved one is close by.

Prepare an environment that is conducive to the practices described in this book. A clean, sacred, thoughtful area or room can be prepared for meditation, visualization, singing and praying. Candles, incense and beautiful pictures can adorn the room. A picture of our loved one can be placed next to images of holy beings that inspire us.

To feel closer, you can, of course, talk to them by phone or video. You, or your children, can create and send artwork or music. Show appreciation and love. Always stay positive.

And finally, let's give the support and love with all that we have. This is all about our devotion and surrender to God or higher being. God or a higher being can continue to support you and your loved one as they pass through their death.

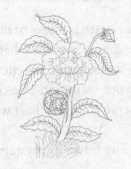

CHAPTER 9

What Can I Do for Myself If I am the Person Dying?

What has passed in this life is ancient history. You are now at the threshold of a beautiful, wondrous and new opportunity.

Death is just as natural as birth. Death is not to be feared. It can be viewed as an opportunity to connect with God, or a higher being. We need to come to a place in our mind where we can accept this.

Focus on the 'prize'—a beautiful transition to the next phase in the cycle of birth, life, death—and do not be distracted by doubts or fears. Through meditation we can learn to stay focused on what is happening now.

Let's not create illusions in our mind.

Reality is that our sense of 'self' is an illusion.

Reality is everything is always changing.

Reality is we die and we go to an afterlife of one kind or another.

Whether you believe in an afterlife or not, why not make your death a celebration?

Why not love yourself like you never have?

Why not encourage your loved ones to support you in the most positive, joyful way they know how?

If you 'know' that your death is weeks or months away, then please practice the prayers and chants provided here on Compassion and Wisdom. Please establish a meditation practice for yourself.

If you can't do it on your own, find a teacher who is supportive.

Feeling stressed? Observe your breath. It will keep you in the present moment.

"The past is history. The future is mystery. The present moment is a gift."

CHAPTER 10

How can we help our loved ones and ourselves immediately after our loved one dies?

When a loved one has passed and is no longer breathing (or death has been verified), being calm, aware and loving can continue to support their consciousness.

From those who have died and returned to their body (NDE), we know that in many cases the deceased can still "hear" what is going on. The consciousness may still be aware and very sensitive, even after death.

For example, agitated crying can still be "heard" and sensed by the deceased. It can impact the deceased's consciousness as they to continue through the bardo.

If this emotion can't be avoided, then best for the bereaved to leave the room until they have calmed down.

Buddhists may leave a body in place, at rest, for a period of time. This is done, once again, to give the consciousness time to acclimate to the bardo with calmness, and to allow Buddhist priests or Lamas to pray and guide the consciousness.

Followers of Tibetan Buddhist schools may leave a body in its place for up to 7 days, according to astrological charts. Everyone is different. Pure Land Buddhists leave a body at rest for 12—24 hours.

Given the practicality and laws of the country, lengthy time periods may not be possible. Best to plan in advance for what is practical and possible. Many leave the body at rest for a few hours. The length of time is not the key factor. How the time is spent during that rest period is of greater importance.

During this time, prayers can be read, poetry can be recited and gentle soft music can be played. It is also very calming and beautiful to have butter lamps or candles lit after the body is deceased—so as not to create any respiratory issues from smoke.

Calm, joyful thoughts about the individual can be of help for both the bereaved and the deceased. Thoughts, speech and actions are all to help the consciousness acclimate, and move on through the bardo in a calm state.

It is our opportunity to wish them peace on their journey, and to encourage their consciousness to move on peacefully to their next phase after death.

Days, or weeks later, consider a celebration event of the deceased's life. It is a celebration of all that the person achieved in their lives, and how they were of benefit to others.

Celebration activities can include donating to the less fortunate, planting a tree in their honor or performing a Life Release.

Life Release is a traditional Buddhist practice of saving the lives of beings that were destined for slaughter. This can be the saving of any animal. It can include purchasing, and then releasing, any animal back into their natural habitat—to be free from slaughter. Examples include fish, crickets, grasshoppers, etc. that were being sold for slaughter.

All activities to benefit others are dedicated to the life of the deceased. This merit will help their consciousness, improve their karma as they navigate the bardo, or move on to their next phase after life.

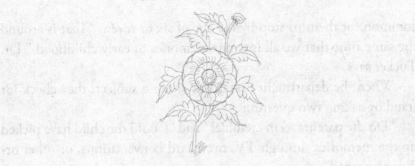

CHAPTER 11

Thoughts about rebirth

University of Virginia School of Medicine (Division of Perceptual Studies) has scientifically documented over 2,500 cases of children—from families of all religions—who have recalled their previous lives in great detail.

The division is lead by Dr. Tucker, a child psychiatrist who now works at the University of Virginia. His department's team of researchers' work includes identifying and validating any claims of rebirth or reincarnation.

The following is summarized and paraphrased from their website—https://med.virginia.edu/perceptual-studies.

Their mission statement reads:

"Division of Perceptual Studies researchers objectively document and rigorously analyze empirical data collected regarding human experiences which suggest that mind and brain may be distinct and separable, *and that consciousness may persist in detectable ways beyond bodily death*."

Many of the children documented by this division were talking about their previous lives when they were two or three years old. It was common for them to stop by the age of six or seven. "That is around the same time that we all lose our memories of early childhood," Dr. Tucker says.

When the department first learns about a subject, they check for fraud by asking two questions:

"Do the parents seem credible?" and "Could the child have picked up the memories through TV, overheard conversations, or other ordinary means?"

Dr. Tucker and his team do additional research to verify authenticity. When they are confident that there is no fraud, they interview the family and the child to get details about the child's previous life.

The researchers then search to find an individual who died; whose life matches the information provided by the child. Verification of the child's memory is key to confirm that the story is not made up in any way.

In addition, almost 20 percent of the children in the University of Virginia cases were born with physical scars or birthmarks, that matched scars or injuries from the person who was identified in the child's previous life.

We understand that the belief in rebirth can be difficult for many of us, but it is good to keep an open mind to the possibilities.

Here are two additional articles on the concept of rebirth:

The Buddhist Teachings on Rebirth
BY LION'S ROAR STAFF| MAY 12, 2018
https://www.lionsroar.com/just-more-of-the-same

Do You Only Live Once? The Evidence for Rebirth
BY SAM LITTLEFAIR| MAY 11, 2018
https://www.lionsroar.com/do-you-only-live-once
Appendix A—Tools for a Happy Life Now and an Auspicious Rebirth Later

May all beings benefit.

54

CHAPTER 12

Essential words of advice for a joyful way of living, peaceful way of dying

Peace in our Mind

What we see—what we hear—what we feel—they are all reflections of our mind.

If we are in a good state of mind, we can see the beauty in what is around us. We can appreciate the things and people in our life. If we are not in a good state of mind, then everything around us is insufficient and lacking.

When we understand our mind, we understand all of life.

We can't change others. We can only change our self.

If we want peace in our lives, then we need to find the peace in our self.

Learn to meditate to be able to live in peace and live in reality without illusion.

The best way to prepare for death is to live a simple life and enjoy it.

The less we have, the fewer problems that we will experience.

Chasing sense objects, or money, will not bring happiness.

Let go of unnecessary material things and petty grievances.

Success and Appreciation

Real success is when we have peace in our home and happiness in our heart. Then we are truly a successful person.

The richest people in the world are still chasing and purchasing things and businesses. Are they enjoying life? Are they satisfied, or do they still want to buy more?

We can have material things, but the real key is to enjoy what we have—now.

If we are rich, it is wonderful because we can share, and give to help others.

In the western world we live in abundance. We need to appreciate it and enjoy it. Enjoy the weather. Enjoy our family. Enjoy our life. It doesn't matter if we are rich or poor—enjoy.

If we want to be happy we need to train ourselves to appreciate what we do have. No need to pine or grasp for what we don't have.

When we appreciate our life, there is no suffering.

Daily Life

When we wake up—create a beautiful motivation for the day. 'I am going to enjoy my work. I am so glad I have a place to sleep. I am glad I have a job to work. I am glad I have a family.'

Eat healthy. Exercise. Speak with your doctor or nutritionist and find out what is best for you. Listen to your body—and learn what is good for you and not good for you.

Practical Planning

We also prepare for death by getting our material and financial affairs in order. This avoids arguments after we are gone. Create a will.

Talk with family members about the dying process, how you feel and what you would like when the time comes.

Put in writing how family or friends can help during the dying process or after death.

Life and death are both an adventure. Prepare and be positive.

APPENDIX

Practices to Develop Compassion and Wisdom

As discussed in Chapter 5, the development of Compassion and Wisdom leads us to a happier life, a peaceful death and an auspicious rebirth. Here are practical methods to integrate these into our lives now:

Practice to Develop Compassion

"If you want others to be happy, practice compassion.
If you want to be happy, practice compassion."
- His Holiness XIV Dalai Lama

Loving-kindness or Compassion Meditation

- Take a few minutes to sit peacefully with your eyes closed and observe your breath as you breathe in and out.
- Allow yourself to breathe naturally, without any modification of the breath.
- For a few minutes, simply observe your breath in its most natural state, as it passes through your nostrils.
- If you find that you are distracted by your thoughts or sounds, no problem; just go back to observing your breath.

Part 1:

When you are calm, recite the following verse to yourself three times, slowly with intention and devotion:

May I be happy.
May I be peaceful.
May I be free from suffering.

Now observe your breath, as you did earlier, for a few moments.

Part 2:

Keeping in mind a loved one or a family member, recite the following verse three times, filling in the loved one's name, slowly with intention and devotion.

May [fill in the name] be happy.
May [fill in the name] be peaceful.
May [fill in the name] be free from suffering.

Now observe your breath, as you did earlier, for a few moments.

Part 3:

Keeping in mind someone you feel neutral about (e.g. the cashier at the grocery store, or someone you don't know that well), recite the verse three times and fill in the person's name. If you don't know their name, it is ok to use a descriptive title (e.g. bank teller):

May [fill in the name] be happy.
May [fill in the name] be peaceful.
May [fill in the name] be free from suffering.

Now observe your breath, as you did earlier, for a few moments.

Part 4:

Bring to mind someone you have difficulty with (e.g. someone you don't care for or find annoying). Recite the verse three times and fill in the person's name:

May [fill in the name] be happy.
May [fill in the name] be peaceful.
May [fill in the name] be free from suffering.

Now observe your breath, as you did earlier, for a few moments.

When done, express to a Higher Being, your teacher or you higher self a sense of gratitude that you have the ability to practice compassion for yourself and others.

How this works:

- When we focus on our breath, we are in the moment.
- Being in the moment automatically stops any habitual thinking about the past and the future.
- When we help others, we feel better.
- When we help ourself, we feel better.
- We are transforming the negative state of mind into positive.
- This trains us to be able to change our state of mind quickly.
- This meditation reduces the attachment to anger—or whatever negative state of mind is being experienced.
- It allows our mind to be more malleable and shows us that our thoughts and emotions are ephemeral.

Practice to Develop Wisdom

"If you wish to make an apple pie from scratch, you must first invent the universe."

- Carl Sagan, Cosmologist

We can use analytical meditation to develop wisdom that helps us understand the 'emptiness of all phenomena', and the reality of our 'self'.

The emptiness of all phenomena means simply that our reality is always changing. No thing is solid and permanent.

By understanding this, and reminding ourselves that everything is always changing, it helps us reduce our grasping and clinging to things that we think are solid and permanent—people, places and experiences.

The grasping and clinging is what causes us suffering.

We typically also view our "self" as a solid permanent being. And, as a result, this makes it difficult for us to be flexible and see others and ourselves with an open mind—without judgment.

We have a view of who we are that is quite fixed—our self-identity. This identity is developed and supported by the stories we tell ourselves, about who we think we are. And when something happens that threatens that view, we can get angry, annoyed or fearful.

By understanding that we are always changing, and that our self doesn't exist in a permanent sense, we can be more flexible with our views of ourselves, others, situations and expectations. We can be more understanding of other people and situations.

Wisdom Realizing Emptiness & No Solid Self:

- Take a few minutes to sit peacefully with your eyes closed; and observe your breath as you breathe in and out.
- Allow yourself to breathe naturally, without any modification of the breath.
- For a few minutes; simply observe your breath in its most natural state, as it passes through your nostrils.
- If you find that you are distracted by your thoughts or sounds, no problem, just go back to observing your breath.

In your mind see a table.

In English, it is described by the word 'table'.

This table is made up of many pieces: a top, legs, glue, nails and varnish.

The legs and top are made up of wood from a tree. Before the tree was cut down it grew as a result of many variables—sunlight, seeds, rain, earth, wind—to name just a few ingredients.

And before it was a tree, it was a seed from another tree, and another tree before that.

What about the nails or the varnish? Those ingredients can also be traced backwards to the people, companies and ingredients that went into their production.

And the people who created the ingredients also came into being from their parents, and their parents before them.

We now see that everything around us—all phenomena—were caused by something that preceded it—and can be traced back to a beginning-less time.

Next time pick another thing, place or person—and go through the same logic. As you go about your day—notice everything around you and apply the same logic.

When you walk around your work or home environment, notice that everything is empty of inherent existence. Everything has a name that refers to a thing that comes together for a time.

Zen teacher Norman Fischer said, "In the end, everything is just a designation. Things have a kind of reality in their being named and conceptualized, but otherwise they actually aren't present."

"In fact, connection is all you find, with no things that are connected. It's the very thoroughness of the connection -- no gaps or lumps in it -- only the constant nexus -- that renders everything void. So everything is empty and connected, or empty because connected. Emptiness is connection."

What about your 'self?

- Take a few minutes to sit peacefully with your eyes closed, and observe your breath as you breathe in and out.

- Allow yourself to breathe naturally, without any modification of the breath.
- For a few minutes simply observe your breath in its most natural state, as it passes through your nostrils.
- If you find that you are distracted by your thoughts or sounds, no problem, just go back to observing your breath.

Read the following and then contemplate each question one at a time:

- Can you identify and define your "self"? Where is it? Can you show it to someone? Is it fixed? Is it permanent?

Close your eyes and contemplate this for a few minutes.

- Are the opinions and views you have of yourself different now then yesterday or a year ago?

Close your eyes and contemplate this for a few minutes.

- What about other people—are they growing or dying—and changing along the way? Might their views, opinions and motivations be changing too?

Close your eyes and contemplate this for a few minutes.

- Consider that we are always changing, and our views of our selves and others are based on an illusion of permanence. The illusion is that we think that our views, and what is around us, are solid and permanent. This is not true.

Close your eyes and contemplate this for a few minutes.

- Thoughts, views, feelings, opinions, motivation and judgment are subject to change from moment to moment—ours and everyone else's. As a result, we would be foolish to judge anyone's motivation, or even trust our own views with great certainty.

As we contemplate this more and more, we will understand that 'reality' is not what we think. It is something more nuanced; always changing, and more illusory than we think.

We can be more open-minded to the views of those around us, and more compassionate to our selves and others.

Close your eyes and contemplate this for a few minutes.

May all beings benefit.

The Tibetan Book of the Dead—A Summary

The *Tibetan Book of the Dead*, composed in the 8th century by the great Buddhist Master Padmasambhava, describes instructions that an accomplished Buddhist Lama uses to guide the dying Buddhist practitioner to liberation, or through the bardos (the post-death states of consciousness) to an auspicious rebirth.

These instructions are also meant to be employed while we are alive and healthy, as part of our daily Buddhist practice. They prepare us to approach death and the bardos and are a road map to liberation.

The *Tibetan Book of the Dead* in the Tibetan language is called *Bardo Thodol*. The direct translation of *Bardo Thodol* is—*Liberation through Hearing in the Intermediate State*.

Why hearing?

Qualified Buddhist Lamas instruct the dying individual by whispering or chanting these prayers, or visualizations, melodiously into their ear.

The Lama has practiced these esoteric, powerful and effective practices for many years, if not lifetimes. In turn, the dying person has ideally practiced these prayers and visualizations throughout their lifetime, and more importantly, developed great devotion and trust in the Lama, who is often their Buddhist teacher.

The Lama is motivated to help reduce suffering of sentient beings. With that strong mindset, the Lama guides the dying person to liberation, or to rebirth.

The *Tibetan Book of the Dead* is read, or recited, by the Lama, and sometimes with monks who join in support of the dying individual. The practices include:

- a description of the 6 bardos that make up the birth-life-death cycle

- an introduction to the ultimate nature of our mind. This phrase can be described as Buddha nature, the primordial aspect of all sentient beings. Other descriptions are: the realization of the emptiness of all phenomena, or the mind that is primordial and radiant (all aware).

- **Shechen Gyaltsab** (1871–1926), a principal lineage holder in Tibetan Buddhism, describes Buddha nature as follows:

  "Buddha-nature is immaculate. It is profound, serene, unfabricated suchness, an uncompounded expanse of luminosity; nonarising, unceasing, primordial peace, spontaneously present nirvana."

Rabjam, Shechen (2007). The Great Medicine: Steps in Meditation on the Enlightened Mind. Boston: Shambhala: p. 4

- a practice where the dying person develops an awareness of the different aspects of their mind.

- a practice for the dying person to help them recognize that everything they see and experience is a reflection of their mind.

- a prostration practice, where prostrations are performed while visualizing Buddhist deities (emanations of enlightened beings) in front of them. The visualization of, and devotion to, these magnificent deities allows the practitioner to purify their own karma, through confession, and expressions of regret for the negative habits they developed during their lifetime.

- a prayer practice where the dying person confesses their negative karma, and resolves not to repeat the actions that caused it.

- a description of how and when the body degrades as it approaches death. This allows the qualified Buddhist Lama to guide the dying person through the practices described here, based on the stages of dying that are taking place.

- a practice that transfers consciousness (negative karma) to a higher being as one dies. By reducing or eliminating negative karma in this way, the dying person can proceed through the bardo to rebirth, without the burden of negative karma.

- a protocol where the Lama can free the dying person from the suffering that all beings experience as they go through cyclic existence (i.e. birth-life-death)

- visualization and recitation practices that help the dying person merge their mind with the mind of enlightenment

- refuge prayers where the dying person expresses their devotion to the 3 Jewels of Buddhism—the Buddha, the Dharma and the Sangha.

- refuge prayers where the dying person expresses their devotion to the Buddhas and Bodhisattvas.

For traditional Buddhist practitioners of Tibetan lineages, these prayers and protocols are chanted to the dying person over many weeks, as they go through the *Bardo of Dying* and the *Bardo of Luminosity*.

May all beings benefit.

About the Authors

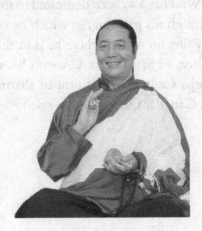

Lama Lhanang

Venerable Lama Lhanang Rinpoche was born in Golok, Amdo northeast of Tibet. As a child, he entered the Thubten Chokor Ling Monastery located in the Gande region, Golok under the guidance of his root teacher Kyabye Orgyen Kusum Lingpa, where in addition to developing a complete monastic education, he trained in the yogi lineage of Anu Yoga.

He was recognized as the rebirth of Ken Rinpoche Damcho, an emanation of Nubchen Namke Nyingpo—one of the 25 disciples of Guru Rinpoche—by the Sang Long Monastery located in eastern Tibet.

He has received teachings from a large number of teachers from the different schools and lineages of Tibetan Buddhism, such as HH Dalai Lama, 4th Dodrupchen Rinpoche, Kyabye Katok Getse Rinpoche, among others.

Lama Lhanang Rinpoche is a teacher of Vajrayana Buddhism, from the Nyingma school of the Longchen Nyingthig lineage. In addition to the instructions of Buddhism, he studied history, astrology, grammar, Tibetan medicine, painting, sculpture, music, theater. All this has led him to share teachings on the proper use of the body, the word and the mind; with the motto: *world peace through inner peace* .

His life in the West has also been dedicated to sharing the teachings of the Buddha through his painting, in which he reflects his relationship with everyday life, no matter where he is in the world.

He currently lives in San Diego, CA with his wife and child. He directs Jigme Lingpa Center, in addition to sharing his teachings in centers in the US, Canada, Europe and Mexico.

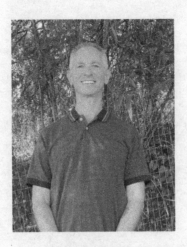

Mordy Levine

Mordy Levine graduated from Brandeis University with a BA. He attended University of Chicago Business School and graduated with an MBA.

Mordy is the creator of the Meditation Pro Series that teaches meditation for different conditions that affect Western civilization (e.g. stress, insomnia, weight issues, smoking). To date, over 950,000 people have learned to meditate through his series of meditation programs.

Mordy is the President of Jigme Lingpa Center, a nonprofit organization led by Lama Lhanang Rinpoche. The center's goal is to generate benefit to all beings through the dissemination of the Buddha's teachings of wisdom and compassion, in order to achieve a sustainable future of peace and harmony for all.

Mordy Levine has been practicing yoga and martial arts for 40 years—almost daily. He also meditates daily.

Mordy holds instructor certifications in Karate, Tai Chi and Yoga.

Mordy and his wife Elizabeth have a son, and live in Rancho Santa Fe with many dogs.

Mardy Levine